CW00641878

ARE YOU FRUITY?

Are You Fruity?

The Little Book of Medicinal Fruits

Walter the Educator

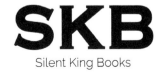
SKB
Silent King Books

Copyright © 2024 by Walter the Educator

All rights reserved. No part of this book may be repro-
duced in any manner whatsoever without written permis-
sion except in the case of brief quotations embodied in
critical articles and reviews.

First Printing, 2024

Disclaimer
This book is for entertainment and informational purposes
only. The author and publisher offer this information without warranties expressed or implied. No matter the
grounds, neither the author nor the publisher will be
accountable for any losses, injuries, or other damages
caused by the reader's use of this book. The use of this
book acknowledges an understanding and acceptance of
this disclaimer.

dedicated to everyone in search of
good health

CONTENTS

ONE

WHY I CREATED THIS BOOK

Creating a book focused on the medicinal properties of various fruits serves as an insightful exploration into the natural world of healing. By delving into the diverse array of fruits and their health benefits, readers can gain a deeper understanding of the potent healing potential found within nature's bounty. This type of publication offers a comprehensive look at the therapeutic attributes of fruits, providing readers with valuable knowledge on how these fruits can positively impact their well-being. Furthermore, this book can serve as a valuable resource for individuals seeking alternative and holistic approaches to wellness, offering a wealth of information on the medicinal properties of fruits and their potential to support a healthy lifestyle. Ultimately, the creation of this book contributes to the ever-expanding body of literature dedicated to promoting holistic health and wellness through the exploration of nature's medicinal treasures.

TWO

AÇAÍ BERRY

Açaí Berry: Known for its high antioxidant content, which can help reduce inflammation and promote heart health.

Consuming Açaí Berry can bestow upon you a plethora of health advantages, ranging from enhanced antioxidant protection to potential heart health reinforcement. These delightful little berries are chockfull of antioxidants, which serve as guardians against oxidative stress, thereby potentially diminishing the risk of chronic diseases and bolstering overall wellbeing. Açaí berries are also brimming with essential nutrients like vitamins A and C, as well as minerals such as calcium and potassium, all contributing to a robust immune system and bone health.

Furthermore, these berries contain healthy fats,

including omega-3 and omega-6 fatty acids, which are conducive to cardiovascular health by aiding in the maintenance of optimal cholesterol levels. Additionally, Açaí berries may assist in regulating blood sugar levels due to their fiber content, potentially reducing the risk of diabetes. Moreover, their anti-inflammatory properties may mitigate inflammation throughout the body, potentially alleviating symptoms of conditions like arthritis. Incorporating Açaí berries into your dietary repertoire can thus be a delicious and nutritious means of fostering vitality and longevity.

THREE

GOJI BERRY

Goji Berry: Contains antioxidants and vitamins that support immune function and may improve skin health.

Eating Goji berries, also known as wolfberries, offers a plethora of health advantages, making it a cherished addition to one's dietary regimen. These small, red-orange berries are revered for their rich nutritional profile and have been a staple in traditional Chinese medicine for centuries. Here are several benefits associated with consuming Goji berries:

1. Antioxidant Powerhouse: Goji berries are brimming with antioxidants, including vitamin C, zeaxanthin, and beta-carotene, which help combat oxidative stress and protect cells from damage caused by free radicals.

2. Boosts Immunity: The high vitamin C content in Goji berries supports a robust immune system, helping the body fend off infections and illnesses.

3. Enhances Eye Health: Goji berries contain zeaxanthin and beta-carotene, which are beneficial for eye health and may help prevent age-related macular degeneration and other vision problems.

4. Supports Heart Health: Consuming Goji berries is linked to improved cardiovascular health due to their ability to lower blood sugar levels, reduce cholesterol, and promote proper circulation.

5. Anti-inflammatory Properties: Goji berries contain various compounds that possess anti-inflammatory properties, aiding in reducing inflammation throughout the body and alleviating symptoms associated with inflammatory conditions.

6. May Aid in Weight Loss: Goji berries are low in calories and rich in fiber, making them a satisfying snack option that can help promote feelings of fullness and aid in weight management.

7. Promotes Skin Health: The antioxidants and vitamins found in Goji berries contribute to healthy, radiant skin by protecting against UV damage, promoting collagen production, and improving overall skin tone and texture.

8. Boosts Energy and Stamina: Goji berries are often touted for their ability to increase energy levels and enhance endurance, making them a popular choice among athletes and individuals seeking a natural

energy boost.

9. Rich Source of Nutrients: In addition to antioxidants and vitamins, Goji berries are packed with essential nutrients such as iron, zinc, and various B vitamins, which are crucial for overall health and well-being.

Incorporating Goji berries into your diet, whether dried, fresh, or in juice form, can provide a wide array of health benefits and contribute to a balanced and nutritious eating plan.

FOUR

ELDERBERRY

Elderberry: Traditionally used to treat colds and flu due to its immune-boosting properties.

Elderberry, a small yet potent fruit harvested from the Sambucus tree, boasts an array of benefits that contribute to overall health and well-being. Rich in antioxidants, elderberries serve as guardians against oxidative stress, bolstering the body's defense against free radicals and potentially reducing the risk of chronic diseases. These vibrant berries also harbor anti-inflammatory properties, soothing bodily inflammation and promoting joint health.

Furthermore, elderberries exhibit immune-boosting prowess, thanks to their high levels of vitamins A and C, as well as flavonoids, which fortify the immune system and aid in fending off infections, particularly respiratory ailments such as colds and flu. Consuming elderberry-based products like syrups, teas, or supplements may help shorten the duration of illnesses and alleviate symptoms.

Moreover, elderberries contribute to cardiovascular health by regulating cholesterol levels and promoting proper blood circulation, thereby reducing the risk of heart disease and stroke. Additionally, these versatile berries support digestive health, facilitating regular bowel movements and alleviating digestive discomfort.

Elderberry consumption also shows promise in promoting skin health, as its antioxidants combat skin damage caused by environmental stressors and aging, fostering a youthful complexion. Some studies even suggest that elderberries possess anti-cancer properties, although further research is needed to substantiate these claims conclusively.

Incorporating elderberries into your diet through various culinary creations or supplements can provide a delicious and nutritious boost to your overall health, offering a natural and flavorful means of enhancing vitality and resilience.

FIVE

CRANBERRY

Cranberry: Well-known for preventing urinary tract infections and promoting urinary health.

Consuming cranberries can yield a plethora of health advantages due to their rich nutrient profile and unique phytochemical composition. These vibrant red berries are renowned for their abundant reserves of antioxidants, particularly flavonoids and polyphenols, which help combat oxidative stress in the body. Incorporating cranberries into your diet can bolster your immune system, as they possess anti-inflammatory and antimicrobial properties, which may aid in preventing urinary tract infections by hindering the adhesion of bacteria to the urinary tract walls.

Moreover, cranberries are a fantastic source of dietary fiber, essential vitamins (such as vitamin C, K, and E), and minerals (including manganese and copper), all of which contribute to digestive health, bone strength, and overall well-being. Additionally, the consumption of cranberries has been associated with promoting cardiovascular health by lowering blood pressure and reducing the risk of heart disease. Furthermore, some studies suggest that the compounds found in cranberries may have anticancer properties, potentially inhibiting the growth and spread of certain cancer cells. Incorporating cranberries into your diet, whether fresh, dried, or in juice form, can thus provide a multitude of health benefits, enhancing both your physical vitality and longevity.

SIX

POMEGRANATE

Pomegranate: Rich in antioxidants, it may help lower blood pressure and reduce the risk of heart disease.

Feasting upon the luscious pomegranate brings forth a plethora of healthful rewards, making it a veritable gem among fruits. Bursting with antioxidants, this crimson marvel bestows upon the consumer a shield against oxidative stress, thwarting the nefarious advances of free radicals and safeguarding cellular integrity. Furthermore, indulging in its succulent arils is akin to imbibing a potion of cardiovascular wellness, as the fruit exerts a salubrious influence on heart health, aiding in the regulation of blood pressure and cholesterol levels.

Rich in potent polyphenols and flavonoids, the

pomegranate wields anti-inflammatory prowess, assuaging bodily inflammation and conferring relief to those beset by maladies such as arthritis. Moreover, this delectable orb harbors a trove of vitamins and minerals, fortifying the immune system and bolstering overall vitality. Delving deeper into its nutritional bounty, one encounters a cornucopia of fiber, promoting digestive regularity and fostering gut health with every delectable bite. Embrace the pomegranate, and revel in its multifaceted bounty, as it bestows upon the discerning epicurean a cornucopia of wellness and vitality.

SEVEN

KIWI

Kiwi: Packed with vitamin C, kiwi can boost the immune system and aid in digestion.

Eating kiwi offers a plethora of advantageous attributes for your health and well-being. Firstly, this fuzzy fruit is bursting with essential nutrients, including vitamin C, vitamin K, vitamin E, folate, and potassium, which are vital for various bodily functions. Incorporating kiwi into your diet can bolster your immune system, aiding in warding off pesky illnesses and infections, while also promoting proper wound healing and collagen production for healthy skin. Moreover, the high fiber content in kiwi supports digestive health by regulating bowel movements and preventing constipation, thus enhancing overall gut function.

Additionally, the potent antioxidants found in kiwi contribute to reducing inflammation and combating oxidative stress, which may lower the risk of chronic diseases like heart disease and cancer. Furthermore, the abundance of phytochemicals and bioactive compounds in kiwi exhibits potential benefits for eye health, cardiovascular health, and even respiratory health. This versatile fruit can be enjoyed in various ways, whether sliced and added to salads, blended into smoothies, or simply eaten on its own for a refreshing and nutritious snack. Overall, embracing kiwi as part of a balanced diet can undoubtedly contribute to optimizing your health and vitality.

EIGHT

BLUEBERRY

Blueberry: Contains anthocyanins, which have been linked to improved brain function and reduced risk of age-related diseases.

Blueberries, those delightful little orbs of sweetness, offer a plethora of benefits that extend far beyond their delicious taste. These tiny fruits pack a powerful punch of nutrition, making them a wonderful addition to any diet.
First and foremost, blueberries are renowned for their high antioxidant content. Antioxidants are compounds that help combat oxidative stress in the body, which can lead to various health issues such as inflammation and chronic diseases. Blueberries are particularly rich in anthocyanins, a type of flavonoid with potent antioxidant properties.

Furthermore, blueberries are excellent for heart health. Consuming them regularly has been linked to lower blood pressure and improved cholesterol levels, reducing the risk of heart disease. Additionally, the fiber content in blueberries supports digestive health by promoting regularity and preventing constipation.

Moreover, these little blue gems are believed to have anti-inflammatory properties, which can help alleviate symptoms of inflammatory conditions such as arthritis. Some studies even suggest that the compounds found in blueberries may have neuroprotective effects, potentially reducing the risk of age-related cognitive decline and improving brain function.

What's more, blueberries are low in calories but high in nutrients, making them an ideal snack for those looking to maintain a healthy weight. They are also versatile and can be enjoyed in numerous ways, whether fresh, frozen, or incorporated into various dishes like smoothies, salads, or desserts.

In conclusion, the benefits of eating blueberries are abundant, ranging from antioxidant and anti-inflammatory properties to heart and brain health support. Incorporating these vibrant berries into your diet can contribute to overall well-being and vitality. So go ahead, indulge in some blueberry goodness and reap the rewards of nature's bounty!

NINE

PINEAPPLE

Pineapple: Contains bromelain, an enzyme with anti-inflammatory properties that may aid digestion and reduce inflammation.

Eating pineapple offers a plethora of advantageous perks for one's well-being. Firstly, this tropical fruit is brimming with essential vitamins and minerals, including vitamin C, manganese, and vitamin B6, fostering a robust immune system and promoting overall health. Its rich antioxidant content aids in combating oxidative stress and reducing the risk of chronic diseases. Moreover, pineapple contains bromelain, an enzyme renowned for its anti-inflammatory properties, which can alleviate inflammation and aid in digestion.

Additionally, the fiber content in pineapple supports digestive health and promotes satiety, aiding in weight management. Incorporating pineapple into your diet may also contribute to improved eye health, bone strength, and enhanced skin complexion. Its deliciously sweet and tangy flavor further enhances culinary experiences, making it a delightful addition to various dishes, beverages, and snacks. Embracing pineapple as part of a balanced diet can undoubtedly amplify both the nutritional value and the gustatory pleasure of your meals.

TEN

PAPAYA

Papaya: Rich in enzymes like papain, which can aid digestion and reduce inflammation.

Consuming papaya offers a plethora of advantageous perks for your health and well-being. This tropical fruit is brimming with essential nutrients, including vitamins A, C, and E, as well as folate, potassium, and magnesium. Indulging in papaya can foster a robust immune system, thanks to its high vitamin C content, which aids in combating infections and bolstering overall immunity.

Furthermore, papaya contains potent antioxidants like beta-carotene and lycopene, which contribute to cellular health and may lower the risk of chronic diseases such as heart disease and certain cancers. Papaya's rich fiber content supports digestive health by promoting regular bowel movements and preventing constipation. Moreover, the enzyme papain found in papaya facilitates digestion by breaking down proteins, potentially easing symptoms of indigestion.

Additionally, papaya possesses anti-inflammatory properties that may alleviate pain and swelling associated with conditions like arthritis. Its low calorie and high water content make it an excellent choice for weight management and hydration.

Furthermore, papaya is renowned for its skin-enhancing properties, promoting a radiant complexion and warding off signs of aging due to its vitamin-rich composition. Embracing papaya as part of a balanced diet can thus contribute to overall vitality and well-being, making it a delectable addition to your culinary repertoire.

ELEVEN

GUAVA

Guava: High in vitamin C and fiber, guava can support immune function and digestive health.

Guava, scientifically known as Psidium guajava, offers a plethora of benefits, ranging from its rich nutrient profile to its medicinal properties. This tropical fruit, native to Central America, Southeast Asia, and Mexico, is renowned for its delicious taste and numerous health advantages.

Firstly, guava is an excellent source of essential vitamins and minerals, including vitamin C, vitamin A, potassium, and dietary fiber. These nutrients contribute to overall health by supporting immune function, promoting healthy vision, regulating blood pressure, and aiding digestion.

Moreover, guava is packed with antioxidants such as

flavonoids, carotenoids, and polyphenols, which help neutralize harmful free radicals in the body, thereby reducing the risk of chronic diseases like cancer, heart disease, and diabetes.

Additionally, guava contains natural compounds like lycopene and quercetin, known for their anti-inflammatory properties. These compounds may help alleviate inflammation, relieve pain, and improve cardiovascular health.

Furthermore, guava is a low-calorie, nutrient-dense fruit, making it an excellent choice for weight management and overall well-being. Its high fiber content promotes satiety, aiding in appetite control and digestion.

Moreover, guava leaves are utilized in traditional medicine for their therapeutic effects. They are believed to possess antimicrobial, anti-diabetic, and anti-inflammatory properties, making them beneficial for treating various ailments such as diarrhea, diabetes, and skin conditions.

In conclusion, incorporating guava into your diet can provide a multitude of health benefits, including immune support, antioxidant protection, anti-inflammatory effects, and digestive health promotion. Embracing this tropical fruit can contribute to a balanced and nutritious diet, enhancing overall vitality and well-being.

TWELVE

MANGO

Mango: Contains compounds like mangiferin, which have antioxidant and anti-inflammatory effects.

Consuming mangoes offers a plethora of advantages, ranging from bolstering overall health to enhancing culinary experiences. These luscious fruits are teeming with essential nutrients like vitamins A, C, and E, as well as minerals such as potassium and magnesium, all of which contribute to robust bodily functions. Mangoes, with their vibrant hues and succulent flesh, not only tantalize taste buds but also promote digestion, thanks to their fiber content, aiding in maintaining gastrointestinal health and preventing constipation.

Furthermore, the antioxidants present in mangoes combat oxidative stress, bolstering the immune system and shielding the body against various ailments. Mangoes are also believed to promote eye health due to their high beta-carotene content, potentially warding off age-related macular degeneration. Moreover, these delectable fruits boast anti-inflammatory properties, potentially mitigating inflammation-related conditions like arthritis. Incorporating mangoes into one's diet can also aid in regulating blood pressure levels and supporting heart health due to their potassium content.

Additionally, mangoes contribute to skin health, imparting a radiant glow and combating signs of aging, owing to their abundance of vitamins and antioxidants. With their exquisite flavor and myriad health benefits, mangoes undoubtedly deserve a prominent place in any well-rounded diet, offering not just gustatory delight but also a bounty of wellness perks.

THIRTEEN

LEMON

Lemon: High in vitamin C, lemons can support immune health and promote detoxification.

Indulging in the consumption of lemons yields a plethora of advantages, ranging from bolstering overall health to enhancing culinary experiences. These zesty citrus fruits are rich in essential nutrients like vitamin C, a potent antioxidant crucial for supporting the immune system and warding off infections.

Additionally, lemons contain flavonoids, compounds known for their anti-inflammatory properties, which may aid in reducing inflammation and lowering the risk of chronic diseases. Incorporating lemon into one's diet can also promote hydration and alkalization, as lemon water is a popular beverage choice for its refreshing taste and purported detoxifying effects.

Furthermore, the citric acid in lemons may aid in digestion by stimulating the production of digestive enzymes and promoting regular bowel movements. Moreover, lemons are believed to contribute to skin health, thanks to their vitamin C content, which supports collagen production and helps maintain a youthful complexion.

Additionally, lemon juice can be used as a natural remedy for various ailments, such as sore throat and indigestion, due to its antibacterial and antiviral properties. Moreover, the aroma of lemons is known to uplift mood and reduce stress, making them a popular choice for aromatherapy and relaxation. With their tangy flavor and myriad health benefits, lemons undoubtedly deserve a prominent place in any well-rounded diet, offering not just gustatory delight but also a bounty of wellness perks.

FOURTEEN

GRAPEFRUIT

Grapefruit: Contains antioxidants like vitamin C and lycopene, which may lower the risk of chronic diseases.

Grapefruits, those tangy and vibrant fruits, pack a plethora of benefits for those who indulge in their juicy goodness. First and foremost, they are a treasure trove of essential vitamins and minerals, including vitamin C, vitamin A, potassium, and dietary fiber, all of which play pivotal roles in maintaining overall health and well-being.

One of the standout qualities of grapefruits is their ability to boost the immune system, thanks to their high vitamin C content, which helps fend off infections and keeps illnesses at bay. Additionally, their rich antioxidant content helps combat free radicals in the body, thus reducing the risk of chronic diseases like heart disease and certain types of cancer.

For those aiming to shed a few pounds or maintain a healthy weight, grapefruits can be a valuable ally. They are low in calories and packed with fiber, making them a satisfying and filling snack that can aid in weight management and promote satiety.

Moreover, grapefruits have been linked to improved heart health, as they can help lower cholesterol levels and regulate blood pressure, ultimately reducing the risk of cardiovascular issues. Their potassium content also supports heart function by assisting in the maintenance of healthy blood pressure levels.

Furthermore, grapefruits may contribute to better digestion and gut health due to their fiber content, which supports regular bowel movements and fosters a healthy digestive system.

In addition to their nutritional benefits, grapefruits can add a burst of flavor and zest to various dishes and beverages, enhancing both taste and nutrition.

However, it's essential to note that grapefruits may interact with certain medications, so individuals taking prescription drugs should consult their healthcare provider before adding grapefruits to their diet to avoid any adverse effects.

In conclusion, the benefits of eating grapefruits are manifold, ranging from immune support and weight management to heart health and digestive wellness, making them a delightful addition to a balanced and nutritious diet.

FIFTEEN

WATERMELON

Watermelon: Rich in lycopene and citrulline, watermelon may help reduce muscle soreness and lower blood pressure.

Watermelon, a luscious fruit brimming with hydration, offers a plethora of health advantages, making it a delightful addition to any diet. Rich in essential vitamins, particularly vitamin C, watermelon aids in bolstering the immune system, fortifying the body's defenses against infections and illnesses.

Furthermore, this succulent fruit contains significant levels of antioxidants, such as lycopene, which may contribute to reducing the risk of chronic diseases like heart disease and certain types of cancer. Moreover, watermelon's high water content and natural electrolytes make it an excellent choice for promoting hydration and replenishing electrolyte levels, particularly during hot weather or after vigorous physical activity. Additionally, its low calorie and fat content make it a guilt-free indulgence for those aiming to maintain or achieve a healthy weight.

Furthermore, watermelon encompasses citrulline, an amino acid linked to enhancing blood flow, potentially supporting cardiovascular health and athletic performance. Lastly, its refreshing and sweet taste makes it a delectable and satisfying treat, providing a burst of natural sweetness without the need for added sugars. Incorporating watermelon into one's dietary regimen can thus contribute to overall well-being, offering a delightful blend of hydration, nutrition, and flavor.

SIXTEEN

DRAGON FRUIT

Dragon Fruit: Contains prebiotics that support gut health and may help control blood sugar levels.

Dragon fruit, also known as pitaya, offers a plethora of benefits that cater to both your taste buds and your health. This exotic fruit, with its vibrant colors and distinct appearance, is not only a feast for the eyes but also a nutritional powerhouse.

First and foremost, dragon fruit is packed with essential vitamins and minerals, including vitamin C, vitamin B, phosphorus, calcium, and iron, among others. These nutrients contribute to overall well-being, supporting immune function, bone health, and energy metabolism.

Moreover, dragon fruit is rich in dietary fiber, which aids in digestion and promotes a healthy gut. Its high fiber content can also help regulate blood sugar levels, making it a beneficial option for individuals managing diabetes or those looking to maintain stable energy levels throughout the day.

Another notable benefit of dragon fruit is its anti-oxidant properties. Antioxidants help combat oxidative stress in the body, reducing the risk of chronic diseases and supporting skin health by neutralizing free radicals.

Additionally, dragon fruit is low in calories and contains no cholesterol, making it a guilt-free option for those watching their weight or looking to improve their heart health. Furthermore, consuming dragon fruit may contribute to hydration due to its high water content, helping to keep you feeling refreshed and revitalized.

In conclusion, incorporating dragon fruit into your diet can be a delicious and nutritious way to enhance your overall health and well-being, providing a range of essential nutrients and antioxidants while offering a unique and delightful culinary experience.

ABOUT THE AUTHOR

Walter the Educator is one of the pseudonyms for Walter Anderson. Formally educated in Chemistry, Business, and Education, he is an educator, an author, a diverse entrepreneur, and he is the son of a disabled war veteran. "Walter the Educator" shares his time between educating and creating. He holds interests and owns several creative projects that entertain, enlighten, enhance, and educate, hoping to inspire and motivate you.

Follow, find new works, and stay up to date
with Walter the Educator™
at WaltertheEducator.com

Milton Keynes UK
Ingram Content Group UK Ltd.
UKHW020738080324
438959UK00014B/500